Stage 3
Kidney Disease Diet

Cookbook for Seniors

Nourishing Recipes to Support Kidney Health and Well-Being.

Judy Kelly

Table of Contents

1. Introduction

Understanding Stage 3 Kidney Disease

Stage 3 kidney disease marks a critical point in the journey of managing chronic kidney disease (CKD). At this stage, the kidneys have sustained moderate damage and are functioning at approximately 30-59% of their normal capacity. While this may sound alarming, it's important to remember that with the right lifestyle changes and medical guidance, it is entirely possible to slow the progression of the disease and maintain a good quality of life.

One of the most crucial aspects of managing stage 3 kidney disease is diet. The foods and drinks you consume play a significant role in maintaining kidney function, controlling symptoms, and preventing further complications. This cookbook is designed to be your go-to resource for creating delicious, kidney-friendly meals that align with your dietary needs.

Importance of Diet in Kidney Health

The kidneys are vital organs responsible for filtering waste and excess fluids from the blood, balancing electrolytes, and regulating blood pressure. When kidney function declines, it becomes harder for the body to manage these tasks effectively. A carefully planned diet can help ease the kidneys' workload by managing the intake of key nutrients such as sodium, potassium, phosphorus, and protein.

Eating a kidney-friendly diet involves:
- Reducing sodium to manage blood pressure and fluid balance.
- Limiting potassium to prevent dangerous buildups in the blood.
- Controlling phosphorus intake to protect bone health.
- Adjusting protein levels to reduce waste products in the blood.

This cookbook will guide you through the process of making these dietary adjustments while still enjoying a variety of tasty and satisfying meals.

How to Use This Cookbook

Navigating dietary restrictions can be challenging, especially if you're used to certain flavors and ingredients. However, with a bit of creativity and knowledge, you can still enjoy a diverse and flavorful diet. This cookbook is structured to help you easily find and prepare meals that fit your kidney health needs.

Each chapter focuses on a specific meal type, from breakfast to dinner, and includes snacks, desserts, and beverages. You'll also find a 7-day meal plan to kickstart your journey, along with practical tips for dining out and managing special occasions. The recipes are designed to be simple and straightforward, with ingredients that are easy to find and prepare.

Here's how to make the most of this cookbook:
- Start with the Basics: Begin by reading the first chapter to understand the fundamentals of a kidney-friendly diet. This foundation will help you make informed choices throughout the rest of the book.
- Explore Recipes: Each recipe includes nutritional information and tips to modify it according to your taste preferences and dietary needs. Feel free to mix and match recipes from different chapters to create balanced meals.
- Plan Ahead: Use the 7-day meal plan as a guide to plan your weekly meals and grocery shopping. This will help you stay on track and make mealtime stress-free.
- Stay Informed: Check out the resources and support section for additional information and guidance on managing kidney disease through diet and lifestyle.

We hope this cookbook becomes a valuable tool in your journey to better kidney health. Remember, every small step you take towards a healthier diet can make a big difference in your overall well-being. Enjoy the process of discovering new recipes and flavors that support your kidney health, and take pride in the positive changes you are making for yourself.

Welcome to the "Stage 3 Kidney Disease Diet Cookbook for Seniors." Let's get started on the path to healthier eating and better living!

2. Chapter 1: The Basics of a Kidney-Friendly Diet

-

Key Nutrients to Monitor

Managing stage 3 kidney disease effectively involves paying close attention to certain nutrients in your diet. Here are the key nutrients you need to monitor:

- Sodium: Excess sodium can lead to high blood pressure and fluid retention, which can further strain your kidneys. Aim to limit sodium intake to less than 2,300 mg per day or as recommended by your healthcare provider. This means avoiding processed foods, salty snacks, and adding less salt to your meals.

- Potassium: While potassium is essential for muscle function and heart health, too much potassium can be harmful for those with kidney disease. High potassium levels can cause irregular heartbeats and muscle weakness. Choose lower-potassium foods such as apples, berries, and green beans, and avoid high-potassium foods like bananas, oranges, and potatoes.

- Phosphorus: High phosphorus levels can lead to bone and heart problems. It's important to limit foods high in phosphorus, such as dairy products, nuts, seeds, and cola beverages. Opt for lower-phosphorus alternatives like rice milk, cream cheese, and fresh fruits and vegetables.

- Protein: Protein is necessary for body repair and maintenance, but too much protein can produce waste that your kidneys have to filter. Focus on moderate protein intake, choosing high-quality sources like lean meats, eggs, and plant-based proteins. Work with your healthcare provider to determine the right amount of protein for you.

Foods to Include

A kidney-friendly diet doesn't have to be bland or restrictive. There are plenty of delicious and nutritious foods you can enjoy:

- Fruits: Apples, berries, cherries, grapes, and peaches are low in potassium and make excellent snacks or additions to meals.
- Vegetables: Cauliflower, bell peppers, lettuce, and cucumbers are great low-potassium options. Try steaming or roasting them for added flavor.
- Grains: White rice, pasta, and bread are lower in phosphorus compared to whole grains. They can be the foundation of many meals.
- Protein Sources: Skinless chicken, fish, and egg whites are good protein choices that are lower in phosphorus and potassium.
- Dairy Alternatives: Opt for rice milk or almond milk instead of cow's milk to reduce phosphorus intake.
- Herbs and Spices: Use fresh herbs and spices to enhance the flavor of your dishes without adding extra sodium.

Foods to Avoid

To manage your kidney disease effectively, it's important to avoid foods that are high in sodium, potassium, and phosphorus:

- Processed Foods: Canned soups, frozen dinners, and deli meats often contain high levels of sodium.
- High-Potassium Foods: Bananas, oranges, tomatoes, and potatoes should be limited or avoided.
- High-Phosphorus Foods: Dairy products, nuts, seeds, and whole grains can contribute to high phosphorus levels.
- Salty Snacks: Chips, pretzels, and salted nuts can increase your sodium intake.
- Dark-Colored Sodas: These beverages often contain high levels of phosphorus.

Tips for Meal Planning and Preparation

Meal planning and preparation are key to maintaining a kidney-friendly diet. Here are some tips to help you get started:

1. Plan Your Meals: Create a weekly meal plan that includes a variety of kidney-friendly foods. This will help you stay on track and make grocery shopping easier.
2. Read Labels: Always check the nutrition labels on packaged foods for sodium, potassium, and phosphorus content.
3. Cook at Home: Preparing meals at home gives you control over the ingredients and allows you to create healthy, delicious dishes.
4. Use Fresh Ingredients: Fresh fruits, vegetables, and meats are usually lower in sodium compared to processed options.
5. Batch Cook: Prepare larger portions of kidney-friendly meals and freeze them in individual servings for quick and easy meals throughout the week.
6. Hydrate Wisely: Drink plenty of water, but be mindful of your fluid intake if your doctor has given you specific guidelines.

By understanding the basics of a kidney-friendly diet and incorporating these tips into your daily routine, you can take an active role in managing your stage 3 kidney disease. In the following chapters, you will find a variety of recipes that are designed to be both delicious and supportive of your kidney health. Let's dive into the world of kidney-friendly cooking and discover how enjoyable and satisfying it can be.

3. Chapter 2: Breakfast Recipes

1. APPLE CINNAMON OATMEAL

Ingredients:
- 1 cup water
- 1/2 cup old-fashioned oats
- 1/2 apple, peeled and diced
- 1/2 tsp ground cinnamon
- 1 tsp honey (optional)

Instructions:
1. Bring water to a boil in a small saucepan.
2. Add oats and diced apple, and reduce heat to a simmer.
3. Cook for 5-7 minutes, stirring occasionally, until oats are tender.
4. Stir in cinnamon and honey, if using.
5. Serve warm.

2. BERRY SMOOTHIE

Ingredients:
- 1/2 cup blueberries
- 1/2 cup strawberries, hulled
- 1/2 cup almond milk
- 1/2 cup plain Greek yogurt
- 1 tbsp honey (optional)
- 1/2 cup ice cubes

Instructions:
1. Combine all ingredients in a blender.
2. Blend until smooth.
3. Pour into a glass and serve immediately.

3. VEGETABLE EGG SCRAMBLE

Ingredients:
- 2 large eggs
- 1/4 cup diced bell pepper
- 1/4 cup diced onion
- 1/4 cup diced zucchini
- 1 tbsp olive oil
- Salt and pepper to taste

Instructions:
1. Heat olive oil in a non-stick skillet over medium heat.
2. Add bell pepper, onion, and zucchini, and sauté until tender.
3. Beat eggs in a bowl and pour over the vegetables.
4. Stir gently until eggs are fully cooked.
5. Season with salt and pepper to taste and serve.

4. CINNAMON RICE PUDDING

Ingredients:
- 1/2 cup cooked white rice
- 1/2 cup almond milk
- 1 tbsp honey
- 1/2 tsp ground cinnamon

Instructions:
1. Combine rice, almond milk, honey, and cinnamon in a saucepan.
2. Cook over medium heat, stirring occasionally, until thickened.
3. Serve warm or chilled.

5. BERRY YOGURT PARFAIT

Ingredients:
- 1/2 cup plain Greek yogurt
- 1/2 cup mixed berries (blueberries, strawberries, raspberries)

- 1 tbsp honey
- 1/4 cup low-sugar granola

Instructions:
1. Layer yogurt, berries, and honey in a glass.
2. Top with granola.
3. Serve immediately.

6. SPINACH AND MUSHROOM OMELET

Ingredients:
- 2 large eggs
- 1/4 cup chopped spinach
- 1/4 cup sliced mushrooms
- 1 tbsp olive oil
- Salt and pepper to taste

Instructions:
1. Heat olive oil in a non-stick skillet over medium heat.
2. Add mushrooms and spinach, and sauté until tender.
3. Beat eggs in a bowl and pour over the vegetables.
4. Cook until the eggs are set, folding the omelet in half.
5. Season with salt and pepper to taste and serve.

7. BANANA PANCAKES

Ingredients:
- 1 ripe banana, mashed
- 2 large eggs
- 1/4 cup almond flour
- 1/2 tsp baking powder
- 1 tsp vanilla extract
- 1 tbsp olive oil

Instructions:
1. In a bowl, combine mashed banana, eggs, almond flour, baking powder, and vanilla extract.
2. Heat olive oil in a non-stick skillet over medium heat.
3. Pour batter into the skillet, forming small pancakes.
4. Cook until bubbles form on the surface, then flip and cook until golden brown.
5. Serve with fresh fruit or a drizzle of honey.

8. STRAWBERRY CHIA PUDDING

Ingredients:
- 1/2 cup almond milk
- 2 tbsp chia seeds
- 1/4 cup diced strawberries
- 1 tbsp honey (optional)

Instructions:
1. In a bowl, mix almond milk, chia seeds, and honey, if using.
2. Stir in diced strawberries.
3. Refrigerate for at least 2 hours or overnight until thickened.
4. Serve chilled.

9. PEACH SMOOTHIE BOWL

Ingredients:
- 1 cup frozen peaches
- 1/2 cup almond milk
- 1/2 cup plain Greek yogurt
- 1 tbsp honey (optional)
- Toppings: fresh peach slices, chia seeds, granola

Instructions:
1. Blend frozen peaches, almond milk, Greek yogurt, and honey until smooth.

2. Pour into a bowl and top with fresh peach slices, chia seeds, and granola.
3. Serve immediately.

10. VEGGIE BREAKFAST BURRITO

Ingredients:
- 1 whole wheat tortilla
- 2 large eggs
- 1/4 cup diced tomatoes
- 1/4 cup diced bell pepper
- 1/4 cup diced onion
- 1 tbsp olive oil
- Salt and pepper to taste

Instructions:
1. Heat olive oil in a non-stick skillet over medium heat.
2. Add tomatoes, bell pepper, and onion, and sauté until tender.
3. Beat eggs in a bowl and pour over the vegetables.
4. Stir gently until eggs are fully cooked.
5. Season with salt and pepper to taste.
6. Spoon the mixture onto the tortilla, roll it up, and serve.

11. BLUEBERRY MUFFINS

Ingredients:
- 1 cup almond flour
- 1/4 cup coconut flour
- 1 tsp baking powder
- 1/2 tsp baking soda
- 2 large eggs
- 1/4 cup honey
- 1/4 cup almond milk
- 1 tsp vanilla extract
- 1 cup fresh blueberries

Instructions:
1. Preheat the oven to 350°F (175°C) and line a muffin tin with paper liners.
2. In a large bowl, combine almond flour, coconut flour, baking powder, and baking soda.
3. In another bowl, whisk eggs, honey, almond milk, and vanilla extract.
4. Pour the wet ingredients into the dry ingredients and mix until combined.
5. Fold in blueberries.
6. Divide the batter among the muffin cups.
7. Bake for 20-25 minutes or until a toothpick inserted into the center comes out clean.
8. Cool before serving.

12. CINNAMON APPLE WAFFLES

Ingredients:
- 1 cup almond flour
- 1/4 cup coconut flour
- 1 tsp baking powder
- 1/2 tsp ground cinnamon
- 2 large eggs
- 1/4 cup unsweetened applesauce
- 1/4 cup almond milk
- 1 tsp vanilla extract

Instructions:
1. Preheat the waffle iron.
2. In a large bowl, mix almond flour, coconut flour, baking powder, and cinnamon.
3. In another bowl, whisk eggs, applesauce, almond milk, and vanilla extract.
4. Pour the wet ingredients into the dry ingredients and mix until combined.
5. Grease the waffle iron with a small amount of oil.

6. Pour the batter into the waffle iron and cook according to the manufacturer's instructions.
7. Serve warm with fresh fruit.

13. AVOCADO TOAST

Ingredients:
- 1 slice whole wheat bread, toasted
- 1/2 ripe avocado
- 1/4 cup diced tomatoes
- 1 tbsp olive oil
- Salt and pepper to taste

Instructions:
1. Mash the avocado in a bowl and spread it over the toasted bread.
2. Top with diced tomatoes and a drizzle of olive oil.
3. Season with salt and pepper to taste.
4. Serve immediately.

14. PEACH YOGURT BOWL

Ingredients:
- 1 cup plain Greek yogurt
- 1/2 cup sliced peaches
- 1 tbsp honey
- 1/4 cup low-sugar granola

Instructions:
1. Spoon Greek yogurt into a bowl.
2. Top with sliced peaches and honey.
3. Sprinkle granola on top.
4. Serve immediately.

15. SPINACH AND TOMATO FRITTATA

Ingredients:
- 2 large eggs
- 1/4 cup chopped spinach
- 1/4 cup diced tomatoes
- 1 tbsp olive oil
- Salt and pepper to taste

Instructions:
1. Preheat the oven to 350°F (175°C).
2. Heat olive oil in an oven-safe skillet over medium heat.
3. Add spinach and tomatoes, and sauté until tender.
4. Beat eggs in a bowl and pour over the vegetables.
5. Cook on the stovetop until the edges are set, then transfer the skillet to the oven.
6. Bake for 10-15 minutes or until the eggs are fully cooked.
7. Season with salt and pepper to taste and serve.

16. MANGO CHIA PUDDING

Ingredients:
- 1/2 cup almond milk
- 2 tbsp chia seeds
- 1/4 cup diced mango
- 1 tbsp honey (optional)

Instructions:
1. In a bowl, mix almond milk, chia seeds, and honey, if using.
2. Stir in diced mango.
3. Refrigerate for at least 2 hours or overnight until thickened.
4. Serve chilled.

17. BREAKFAST QUINOA BOWL

Ingredients:
- 1/2 cup cooked quinoa
- 1/2 cup almond milk
- 1/4 cup mixed berries (blueberries, strawberries, raspberries)
- 1 tbsp honey (optional)
- 1/2 tsp ground cinnamon

Instructions:
1. In a bowl, combine cooked quinoa and almond milk.
2. Top with mixed berries.
3. Drizzle with honey, if using, and sprinkle with cinnamon.
4. Serve immediately.

18. EGG MUFFINS

Ingredients:
- 4 large eggs
- 1/4 cup diced bell pepper
- 1/4 cup diced onion
- 1/4 cup chopped spinach
- 1/4 cup diced tomatoes
- Salt and pepper to taste

Instructions:
1. Preheat the oven to 350°F (175°C).
2. Grease a muffin tin with non-stick spray.
3. In a bowl, beat the eggs and season with salt and pepper.
4. Divide the vegetables evenly among the muffin cups.
5. Pour the beaten eggs over the vegetables.
6. Bake for 15-20 minutes or until the eggs are fully set.
7. Cool slightly before serving.

19. STRAWBERRY BANANA SMOOTHIE

Ingredients:
- 1/2 cup strawberries, hulled
- 1/2 banana
- 1/2 cup almond milk
- 1/2 cup plain Greek yogurt
- 1 tbsp honey (optional)
- 1/2 cup ice cubes

Instructions:
1. Combine all ingredients in a blender.
2. Blend until smooth.
3. Pour into a glass and serve immediately.

20. APPLE WALNUT OATMEAL

Ingredients:
- 1 cup water
- 1/2 cup old-fashioned oats
- 1/2 apple, peeled and diced
- 1/4 cup chopped walnuts
- 1/2 tsp ground cinnamon
- 1 tbsp honey (optional)

Instructions:
1. Bring water to a boil in a small saucepan.
2. Add oats and diced apple, and reduce heat to a simmer.
3. Cook for 5-7 minutes, stirring occasionally, until oats are tender.
4. Stir in chopped walnuts, cinnamon, and honey, if using.
5. Serve warm.

4. Chapter 3: Lunch Recipes

1. GRILLED CHICKEN SALAD

Ingredients:
- 1 boneless, skinless chicken breast
- 1 tbsp olive oil
- Salt and pepper to taste
- 2 cups mixed greens (lettuce, spinach, arugula)
- 1/2 cup cherry tomatoes, halved
- 1/4 cup cucumber, sliced
- 1/4 cup red bell pepper, sliced
- 2 tbsp balsamic vinaigrette

Instructions:
1. Preheat the grill to medium-high heat.
2. Brush the chicken breast with olive oil and season with salt and pepper.
3. Grill the chicken for 6-7 minutes per side, or until fully cooked.
4. Let the chicken rest for 5 minutes, then slice thinly.
5. In a large bowl, combine mixed greens, cherry tomatoes, cucumber, and red bell pepper.
6. Top the salad with sliced chicken and drizzle with balsamic vinaigrette.
7. Serve immediately.

2. QUINOA AND VEGETABLE STIR-FRY

Ingredients:
- 1 cup cooked quinoa
- 1/2 cup broccoli florets
- 1/2 cup sliced bell peppers
- 1/2 cup snap peas
- 1/4 cup diced onion
- 1 tbsp olive oil
- 2 tbsp low-sodium soy sauce
- 1 tsp sesame oil

- 1 tsp minced garlic
- 1 tsp minced ginger

Instructions:
1. Heat olive oil in a large skillet over medium-high heat.
2. Add onion, garlic, and ginger, and sauté for 2-3 minutes.
3. Add broccoli, bell peppers, and snap peas, and stir-fry for 5-7 minutes until vegetables are tender.
4. Stir in cooked quinoa, soy sauce, and sesame oil, and cook for another 2 minutes.
5. Serve warm.

3. TURKEY AND AVOCADO WRAP

Ingredients:
- 1 whole wheat tortilla
- 4 slices deli turkey breast (low sodium)
- 1/2 ripe avocado, sliced
- 1/2 cup mixed greens (lettuce, spinach)
- 1/4 cup shredded carrots
- 1 tbsp hummus

Instructions:
1. Lay the tortilla flat and spread hummus evenly over it.
2. Layer turkey slices, avocado, mixed greens, and shredded carrots.
3. Roll up the tortilla tightly and slice in half.
4. Serve immediately.

4. LENTIL AND VEGETABLE SOUP

Ingredients:
- 1 cup dried lentils, rinsed
- 1 tbsp olive oil
- 1/2 cup diced onion
- 1/2 cup diced celery

- 1/2 cup diced carrots
- 1/2 cup diced tomatoes
- 4 cups low-sodium vegetable broth
- 1 tsp dried thyme
- 1 tsp dried basil
- Salt and pepper to taste

Instructions:
1. Heat olive oil in a large pot over medium heat.
2. Add onion, celery, and carrots, and sauté for 5 minutes until vegetables are softened.
3. Stir in lentils, tomatoes, vegetable broth, thyme, and basil.
4. Bring to a boil, then reduce heat and simmer for 30-35 minutes until lentils are tender.
5. Season with salt and pepper to taste.
6. Serve hot.

5. CHICKEN AND VEGETABLE KEBABS

Ingredients:
- 2 boneless, skinless chicken breasts, cut into cubes
- 1/2 cup cherry tomatoes
- 1/2 cup bell peppers, cut into chunks
- 1/2 cup zucchini, sliced
- 1/4 cup red onion, cut into chunks
- 2 tbsp olive oil
- 1 tbsp lemon juice
- 1 tsp dried oregano
- Salt and pepper to taste

Instructions:
1. Preheat the grill to medium-high heat.
2. In a bowl, combine olive oil, lemon juice, oregano, salt, and pepper.
3. Add chicken and vegetables to the bowl and toss to coat.
4. Thread chicken and vegetables onto skewers.

5. Grill kebabs for 10-12 minutes, turning occasionally, until chicken is fully cooked.
6. Serve immediately.

6. TUNA SALAD LETTUCE WRAPS

Ingredients:
- 1 can (5 oz) tuna in water, drained
- 1/4 cup plain Greek yogurt
- 1 tbsp lemon juice
- 1/4 cup diced celery
- 1/4 cup diced red onion
- 1/4 cup diced bell pepper
- Salt and pepper to taste
- 4 large lettuce leaves

Instructions:
1. In a bowl, combine tuna, Greek yogurt, lemon juice, celery, red onion, and bell pepper.
2. Season with salt and pepper to taste.
3. Spoon the tuna mixture onto lettuce leaves and roll up.
4. Serve immediately.

7. VEGETABLE STUFFED PEPPERS

Ingredients:
- 2 bell peppers, halved and seeded
- 1 cup cooked quinoa
- 1/2 cup diced tomatoes
- 1/4 cup diced zucchini
- 1/4 cup diced onion
- 1 tbsp olive oil
- 1 tsp dried basil
- Salt and pepper to taste

Instructions:
1. Preheat the oven to 375°F (190°C).
2. Heat olive oil in a skillet over medium heat.
3. Add onion and zucchini, and sauté until tender.
4. Stir in quinoa, tomatoes, basil, salt, and pepper.
5. Spoon the mixture into the bell pepper halves.
6. Place stuffed peppers in a baking dish and cover with foil.
7. Bake for 25-30 minutes until peppers are tender.
8. Serve warm.

8. SHRIMP AND VEGETABLE STIR-FRY

Ingredients:
- 1/2 lb shrimp, peeled and deveined
- 1/2 cup broccoli florets
- 1/2 cup sliced bell peppers
- 1/2 cup snap peas
- 1/4 cup diced onion
- 1 tbsp olive oil
- 2 tbsp low-sodium soy sauce
- 1 tsp sesame oil
- 1 tsp minced garlic
- 1 tsp minced ginger

Instructions:
1. Heat olive oil in a large skillet over medium-high heat.
2. Add onion, garlic, and ginger, and sauté for 2-3 minutes.
3. Add shrimp and cook until pink and opaque.
4. Remove shrimp from the skillet and set aside.
5. Add broccoli, bell peppers, and snap peas to the skillet, and stir-fry for 5-7 minutes until vegetables are tender.
6. Return shrimp to the skillet and stir in soy sauce and sesame oil.
7. Cook for another 2 minutes.
8. Serve warm.

9. TURKEY BURGER WITH AVOCADO

Ingredients:
- 1 lb ground turkey
- 1/4 cup diced onion
- 1/4 cup breadcrumbs
- 1 egg
- 1/2 tsp garlic powder
- Salt and pepper to taste
- 1 avocado, sliced
- 4 whole wheat burger buns
- Lettuce and tomato slices

Instructions:
1. In a bowl, combine ground turkey, onion, breadcrumbs, egg, garlic powder, salt, and pepper.
2. Form the mixture into 4 patties.
3. Heat a skillet or grill over medium-high heat.
4. Cook the patties for 5-6 minutes per side, or until fully cooked.
5. Serve the turkey burgers on whole wheat buns with lettuce, tomato, and avocado slices.

10. ROASTED VEGETABLE QUINOA SALAD

Ingredients:
- 1 cup cooked quinoa
- 1/2 cup roasted sweet potatoes
- 1/2 cup roasted bell peppers
- 1/2 cup roasted zucchini
- 1/4 cup diced red onion
- 2 tbsp olive oil
- 1 tbsp balsamic vinegar
- Salt and pepper to taste

Instructions:

1. Preheat the oven to 400°F (200°C).

2. Toss sweet potatoes, bell peppers, zucchini, and red onion with 1 tbsp olive oil.

3. Spread the vegetables on a baking sheet and roast for 20-25 minutes, or until tender.

4. In a large bowl, combine cooked quinoa and roasted vegetables.

5. Drizzle with the remaining olive oil and balsamic vinegar.

6. Season with salt and pepper to taste.

7. Serve warm or chilled.

11. CHICKEN AND AVOCADO SALAD

Ingredients:

- 1 boneless, skinless chicken breast
- 1 tbsp olive oil
- Salt and pepper to taste
- 2 cups mixed greens (lettuce, spinach, arugula)
- 1/2 avocado, sliced
- 1/4 cup cherry tomatoes, halved
- 1/4 cup cucumber, sliced
- 2 tbsp lemon vinaigrette

Instructions:

1. Preheat the grill to medium-high heat.

2. Brush the chicken breast with olive oil and season with salt and pepper.

3. Grill the chicken for 6-7 minutes per side, or until fully cooked.

4. Let the chicken rest for 5 minutes, then slice thinly.

5. In a large bowl, combine mixed greens, avocado, cherry tomatoes, and cucumber.

6. Top the salad with sliced chicken and drizzle with lemon vinaigrette.

12. SPINACH AND FETA STUFFED CHICKEN BREAST

Ingredients:
- 2 boneless, skinless chicken breasts
- 1/2 cup fresh spinach, chopped
- 1/4 cup crumbled feta cheese
- 1 tbsp olive oil
- Salt and pepper to taste

Instructions:
1. Preheat the oven to 375°F (190°C).
2. Cut a pocket into each chicken breast and season with salt and pepper.
3. In a small bowl, mix spinach and feta cheese.
4. Stuff the spinach and feta mixture into the chicken pockets.
5. Secure the openings with toothpicks.
6. Heat olive oil in an oven-safe skillet over medium heat.
7. Sear the chicken breasts for 2-3 minutes per side until browned.
8. Transfer the skillet to the oven and bake for 20-25 minutes, or until the chicken is fully cooked.
9. Remove toothpicks before serving.

13. GREEK YOGURT CHICKEN SALAD

Ingredients:
- 2 cups cooked, shredded chicken breast
- 1/2 cup plain Greek yogurt
- 1 tbsp lemon juice
- 1/4 cup diced celery
- 1/4 cup diced red onion
- 1/4 cup diced red bell pepper
- Salt and pepper to taste
- 4 large lettuce leaves

Instructions:
1. In a bowl, combine shredded chicken, Greek yogurt, lemon juice, celery, red onion, and red bell pepper.
2. Season with salt and pepper to taste.
3. Spoon the chicken mixture onto lettuce leaves and roll up.
4. Serve immediately.

14. VEGETABLE AND HUMMUS WRAP

Ingredients:
- 1 whole wheat tortilla
- 1/4 cup hummus
- 1/2 cup mixed greens (lettuce, spinach, arugula)
- 1/4 cup shredded carrots
- 1/4 cup sliced cucumber
- 1/4 cup sliced bell pepper

Instructions:
1. Lay the tortilla flat and spread hummus evenly over it.
2. Layer mixed greens, shredded carrots, cucumber, and bell pepper.
3. Roll up the tortilla tightly and slice in half.
4. Serve immediately.

15. SALMON AND AVOCADO SALAD

Ingredients:
- 4 oz cooked salmon, flaked
- 1/2 avocado, sliced
- 2 cups mixed greens (lettuce, spinach, arugula)
- 1/4 cup cherry tomatoes, halved
- 1/4 cup cucumber, sliced
- 2 tbsp lemon vinaigrette

Instructions:
1. In a large bowl, combine mixed greens, cherry tomatoes, and cucumber.

2. Top with flaked salmon and avocado slices.
3. Drizzle with lemon vinaigrette.
4. Serve immediately.

16. ROASTED CHICKPEA AND VEGETABLE SALAD

Ingredients:
- 1 can (15 oz) chickpeas, drained and rinsed
- 1/2 cup diced zucchini
- 1/2 cup diced bell peppers
- 1/4 cup diced red onion
- 2 tbsp olive oil
- 1 tsp ground cumin
- 1 tsp ground paprika
- Salt and pepper to taste
- 2 cups mixed greens (lettuce, spinach, arugula)
- 2 tbsp lemon vinaigrette

Instructions:
1. Preheat the oven to 400°F (200°C).
2. Toss chickpeas, zucchini, bell peppers, and red onion with olive oil, cumin, paprika, salt, and pepper.
3. Spread the mixture on a baking sheet and roast for 20-25 minutes, or until vegetables are tender.
4. In a large bowl, combine mixed greens and roasted chickpea mixture.
5. Drizzle with lemon vinaigrette.
6. Serve warm or chilled.

17. CHICKEN AND VEGETABLE SOUP

Ingredients:
- 1 tbsp olive oil
- 1/2 cup diced onion
- 1/2 cup diced celery
- 1/2 cup diced carrots

- 2 cups diced cooked chicken breast
- 4 cups low-sodium chicken broth
- 1 cup diced tomatoes
- 1/2 cup diced zucchini
- 1 tsp dried thyme
- Salt and pepper to taste

Instructions:
1. Heat olive oil in a large pot over medium heat.
2. Add onion, celery, and carrots, and sauté for 5 minutes until vegetables are softened.
3. Stir in chicken, chicken broth, tomatoes, zucchini, thyme, salt, and pepper.
4. Bring to a boil, then reduce heat and simmer for 20-25 minutes until vegetables are tender.
5. Serve hot.

18. TURKEY AND SPINACH STUFFED SWEET POTATOES

Ingredients:
- 2 medium sweet potatoes
- 1/2 lb ground turkey
- 1/2 cup fresh spinach, chopped
- 1/4 cup diced onion
- 1 tbsp olive oil
- 1/2 tsp garlic powder
- Salt and pepper to taste

Instructions:
1. Preheat the oven to 400°F (200°C).
2. Pierce sweet potatoes with a fork and bake for 45-50 minutes, or until tender.
3. In a skillet, heat olive oil over medium heat.
4. Add onion and ground turkey, cooking until turkey is browned.

5. Stir in spinach, garlic powder, salt, and pepper, and cook until spinach is wilted.
6. Slice baked sweet potatoes open and stuff with turkey mixture.
7. Serve immediately.

19. BAKED COD WITH HERBS

Ingredients:
- 2 cod filets
- 1 tbsp olive oil
- 1 tsp dried thyme
- 1 tsp dried oregano
- Salt and pepper to taste
- Lemon wedges for serving

Instructions:
1. Preheat the oven to 375°F (190°C).
2. Place cod filets on a baking sheet and drizzle with olive oil.
3. Sprinkle it with thyme, oregano, salt, and pepper.
4. Bake for 15-20 minutes, or until the fish is flaky and cooked through.
5. Serve with lemon wedges.

20. TOFU AND VEGETABLE STIR-FRY

Ingredients:
- 1 block firm tofu, drained and cubed
- 1/2 cup broccoli florets
- 1/2 cup sliced bell peppers
- 1/2 cup snap peas
- 1/4 cup diced onion
- 1 tbsp olive oil
- 2 tbsp low-sodium soy sauce
- 1 tsp sesame oil
- 1 tsp minced garlic
- 1 tsp minced ginger

Instructions:

1. Heat olive oil in a large skillet over medium-high heat.

2. Add onion, garlic, and ginger, and sauté for 2-3 minutes.

3. Add tofu and cook until lightly browned on all sides.

4. Remove tofu from the skillet and set aside.

5. Add broccoli, bell peppers, and snap peas to the skillet, and stir-fry for 5-7 minutes until vegetables are tender.

6. Return tofu to the skillet and stir in soy sauce and sesame oil.

7. Cook for another 2 minutes.

8. Serve warm.

5. Chapter 4: Dinner Recipes

- 1. BAKED SALMON WITH ASPARAGUS

Ingredients:
- 2 salmon filets
- 1 bunch asparagus, trimmed
- 2 tbsp olive oil
- 1 lemon, sliced
- 1 tsp dried dill
- Salt and pepper to taste

Instructions:
1. Preheat the oven to 375°F (190°C).
2. Place salmon filets and asparagus on a baking sheet.
3. Drizzle with olive oil and sprinkle with dill, salt, and pepper.
4. Top the salmon with lemon slices.
5. Bake for 20-25 minutes, or until salmon is cooked through and asparagus is tender.
6. Serve immediately.

2. CHICKEN AND VEGETABLE STIR-FRY

Ingredients:
- 2 boneless, skinless chicken breasts, sliced
- 1/2 cup broccoli florets
- 1/2 cup sliced bell peppers
- 1/2 cup snap peas
- 1/4 cup diced onion
- 1 tbsp olive oil
- 2 tbsp low-sodium soy sauce
- 1 tsp sesame oil
- 1 tsp minced garlic
- 1 tsp minced ginger

Instructions:
1. Heat olive oil in a large skillet over medium-high heat.
2. Add onion, garlic, and ginger, and sauté for 2-3 minutes.
3. Add chicken and cook until no longer pink.
4. Add broccoli, bell peppers, and snap peas, and stir-fry for 5-7 minutes until vegetables are tender.
5. Stir in soy sauce and sesame oil, and cook for another 2 minutes.
6. Serve warm.

3. QUINOA-STUFFED BELL PEPPERS

Ingredients:
- 4 bell peppers, halved and seeded
- 1 cup cooked quinoa
- 1/2 cup black beans, rinsed and drained
- 1/2 cup corn kernels
- 1/4 cup diced tomatoes
- 1/4 cup diced onion
- 1 tbsp olive oil
- 1 tsp ground cumin
- 1 tsp chili powder
- Salt and pepper to taste

Instructions:
1. Preheat the oven to 375°F (190°C).
2. Heat olive oil in a skillet over medium heat.
3. Add onion and cook until softened.
4. Stir in quinoa, black beans, corn, tomatoes, cumin, chili powder, salt, and pepper.
5. Spoon the mixture into the bell pepper halves.
6. Place stuffed peppers in a baking dish and cover with foil.
7. Bake for 25-30 minutes until peppers are tender.
8. Serve warm.

4. TURKEY MEATBALLS WITH ZUCCHINI NOODLES

Ingredients:
- 1 lb ground turkey
- 1/4 cup breadcrumbs
- 1 egg
- 1/4 cup grated Parmesan cheese
- 1 tsp garlic powder
- 1 tsp dried oregano
- Salt and pepper to taste
- 2 large zucchinis, spiralized
- 1 tbsp olive oil
- 1 cup marinara sauce

Instructions:
1. Preheat the oven to 375°F (190°C).
2. In a bowl, combine ground turkey, breadcrumbs, egg, Parmesan cheese, garlic powder, oregano, salt, and pepper.
3. Form the mixture into meatballs and place on a baking sheet.
4. Bake for 20-25 minutes, or until meatballs are fully cooked.
5. Meanwhile, heat olive oil in a skillet over medium heat.
6. Add zucchini noodles and sauté for 2-3 minutes until tender.
7. Serve meatballs over zucchini noodles, topped with marinara sauce.

5. BAKED CHICKEN AND VEGETABLES

Ingredients:
- 2 boneless, skinless chicken breasts
- 1 cup baby carrots
- 1 cup Brussels sprouts, halved
- 1 cup diced sweet potatoes
- 2 tbsp olive oil
- 1 tsp dried rosemary
- 1 tsp dried thyme
- Salt and pepper to taste

Instructions:
1. Preheat the oven to 400°F (200°C).
2. Place chicken breasts and vegetables on a baking sheet.
3. Drizzle with olive oil and sprinkle with rosemary, thyme, salt, and pepper.
4. Toss to coat evenly.
5. Bake for 25-30 minutes, or until chicken is fully cooked and vegetables are tender.
6. Serve warm.

6. SHRIMP AND VEGETABLE SKEWERS

Ingredients:
- 1/2 lb shrimp, peeled and deveined
- 1/2 cup cherry tomatoes
- 1/2 cup bell peppers, cut into chunks
- 1/2 cup zucchini, sliced
- 1/4 cup red onion, cut into chunks
- 2 tbsp olive oil
- 1 tbsp lemon juice
- 1 tsp dried oregano
- Salt and pepper to taste

Instructions:
1. Preheat the grill to medium-high heat.
2. In a bowl, combine olive oil, lemon juice, oregano, salt, and pepper.
3. Add shrimp and vegetables to the bowl and toss to coat.
4. Thread shrimp and vegetables onto skewers.
5. Grill skewers for 10-12 minutes, turning occasionally, until shrimp is cooked through.
6. Serve immediately.

7. LEMON HERB BAKED COD

Ingredients:
- 2 cod filets
- 1 tbsp olive oil
- 1 lemon, sliced
- 1 tsp dried dill
- 1 tsp dried parsley
- Salt and pepper to taste

Instructions:
1. Preheat the oven to 375°F (190°C).
2. Place cod filets on a baking sheet and drizzle with olive oil.
3. Sprinkle it with dill, parsley, salt, and pepper.
4. Top the cod with lemon slices.
5. Bake for 15-20 minutes, or until the fish is flaky and cooked through.
6. Serve with lemon wedges.

8. SPINACH AND FETA STUFFED CHICKEN

Ingredients:
- 2 boneless, skinless chicken breasts
- 1/2 cup fresh spinach, chopped
- 1/4 cup crumbled feta cheese
- 1 tbsp olive oil
- Salt and pepper to taste

Instructions:
1. Preheat the oven to 375°F (190°C).
2. Cut a pocket into each chicken breast and season with salt and pepper.
3. In a small bowl, mix spinach and feta cheese.
4. Stuff the spinach and feta mixture into the chicken pockets.
5. Secure the openings with toothpicks.
6. Heat olive oil in an oven-safe skillet over medium heat.
7. Sear the chicken breasts for 2-3 minutes per side until browned.

8. Transfer the skillet to the oven and bake for 20-25 minutes, or until the chicken is fully cooked.
9. Remove toothpicks before serving.

9. ROASTED VEGETABLE AND QUINOA BOWL

Ingredients:
- 1 cup cooked quinoa
- 1/2 cup roasted sweet potatoes
- 1/2 cup roasted bell peppers
- 1/2 cup roasted zucchini
- 1/4 cup diced red onion
- 2 tbsp olive oil
- 1 tbsp balsamic vinegar
- Salt and pepper to taste

Instructions:
1. Preheat the oven to 400°F (200°C).
2. Toss sweet potatoes, bell peppers, zucchini, and red onion with 1 tbsp olive oil.
3. Spread the vegetables on a baking sheet and roast for 20-25 minutes, or until tender.
4. In a large bowl, combine cooked quinoa and roasted vegetables.
5. Drizzle with the remaining olive oil and balsamic vinegar.
6. Season with salt and pepper to taste.
7. Serve warm or chilled.

10. GARLIC BUTTER SHRIMP

Ingredients:
- 1/2 lb shrimp, peeled and deveined
- 2 tbsp unsalted butter
- 3 cloves garlic, minced
- 1 tbsp lemon juice
- 1/4 cup fresh parsley, chopped

- Salt and pepper to taste

Instructions:
1. Heat butter in a large skillet over medium heat.
2. Add garlic and sauté for 1-2 minutes until fragrant.
3. Add shrimp and cook until pink and opaque.
4. Stir in lemon juice, parsley, salt, and pepper.
5. Serve immediately.

11. TURKEY AND VEGETABLE CHILI

Ingredients:
- 1 lb ground turkey
- 1 tbsp olive oil
- 1/2 cup diced onion
- 1/2 cup diced bell peppers
- 1/2 cup diced zucchini
- 1 cup diced tomatoes
- 1 cup black beans, rinsed and drained
- 2 cups low-sodium chicken broth
- 1 tbsp chili powder
- 1 tsp ground cumin
- 1 tsp dried oregano
- Salt and pepper to taste

Instructions:
1. Heat olive oil in a large pot over medium heat.
2. Add onion and bell peppers, and sauté until softened.
3. Add ground turkey and cook until browned.
4. Stir in zucchini, tomatoes, black beans, chicken broth, chili powder, cumin, oregano, salt, and pepper.
5. Bring to a boil, then reduce heat and simmer for 25-30 minutes.
6. Serve hot.

12. BAKED EGGPLANT PARMESAN

Ingredients:
- 1 large eggplant, sliced into 12. BAKED EGGPLANT PARMESAN

Ingredients:
- 1 large eggplant, sliced into 1/2-inch rounds
- 1 cup whole wheat breadcrumbs
- 1/2 cup grated Parmesan cheese
- 2 eggs, beaten
- 2 cups marinara sauce
- 1 cup shredded mozzarella cheese
- 1 tbsp olive oil
- Salt and pepper to taste

Instructions:
1. Preheat the oven to 375°F (190°C).
2. Sprinkle eggplant slices with salt and let sit for 15 minutes to draw out moisture. Pat dry with paper towels.
3. In a shallow dish, combine breadcrumbs and Parmesan cheese.
4. Dip each eggplant slice in beaten eggs, then coat with the breadcrumb mixture.
5. Place the breaded eggplant slices on a baking sheet and drizzle with olive oil.
6. Bake for 20 minutes, flipping halfway through, until golden brown.
7. Spread 1/2 cup of marinara sauce in a baking dish.
8. Layer half of the eggplant slices over the sauce.
9. Top with 1/2 cup of marinara sauce and 1/2 cup of mozzarella cheese.
10. Repeat the layers with the remaining eggplant, sauce, and cheese.
11. Bake for 20-25 minutes, or until the cheese is melted and bubbly.
12. Serve hot.

13. LEMON GARLIC ROASTED CHICKEN

Ingredients:
- 1 whole chicken (about 4 lbs)
- 1 lemon, halved
- 4 cloves garlic, minced
- 2 tbsp olive oil
- 1 tbsp fresh rosemary, chopped
- 1 tbsp fresh thyme, chopped
- Salt and pepper to taste

Instructions:
1. Preheat the oven to 425°F (220°C).
2. Pat the chicken dry with paper towels.
3. Rub the chicken with olive oil, garlic, rosemary, thyme, salt, and pepper.
4. Place the lemon halves inside the chicken cavity.
5. Place the chicken in a roasting pan.
6. Roast for 1 hour and 15 minutes, or until the internal temperature reaches 165°F (74°C).
7. Let the chicken rest for 10 minutes before carving.
8. Serve with pan juices.

14. VEGETABLE LASAGNA

Ingredients:
- 9 lasagna noodles
- 2 cups ricotta cheese
- 1 cup shredded mozzarella cheese
- 1/2 cup grated Parmesan cheese
- 2 cups spinach, chopped
- 1 zucchini, sliced
- 1 yellow squash, sliced
- 1 cup mushrooms, sliced
- 4 cups marinara sauce
- 1 tbsp olive oil

- Salt and pepper to taste

Instructions:
1. Preheat the oven to 375°F (190°C).
2. Cook lasagna noodles according to package instructions. Drain and set aside.
3. In a skillet, heat olive oil over medium heat.
4. Add zucchini, squash, and mushrooms, and sauté until tender. Season with salt and pepper.
5. In a mixing bowl, combine ricotta cheese, spinach, and 1/4 cup of Parmesan cheese.
6. Spread 1/2 cup of marinara sauce on the bottom of a baking dish.
7. Layer 3 lasagna noodles over the sauce.
8. Spread half of the ricotta mixture over the noodles.
9. Top with half of the sautéed vegetables and 1 cup of marinara sauce.
10. Repeat layers with the remaining noodles, ricotta mixture, vegetables, and sauce.
11. Top with shredded mozzarella and the remaining Parmesan cheese.
12. Cover with foil and bake for 30 minutes.
13. Remove the foil and bake for an additional 15 minutes, or until the cheese is melted and bubbly.
14. Let the lasagna rest for 10 minutes before slicing and serving.

15. BEEF AND BROCCOLI STIR-FRY

Ingredients:
- 1 lb flank steak, thinly sliced
- 2 cups broccoli florets
- 1/2 cup sliced bell peppers
- 1/4 cup sliced onion
- 3 cloves garlic, minced
- 2 tbsp olive oil
- 1/4 cup low-sodium soy sauce
- 1 tbsp oyster sauce
- 1 tbsp cornstarch mixed with 2 tbsp water

- 1 tsp sesame oil

Instructions:
1. Heat 1 tbsp of olive oil in a large skillet over medium-high heat.
2. Add the steak and cook until browned. Remove from the skillet and set aside.
3. Add the remaining olive oil to the skillet.
4. Add garlic, broccoli, bell peppers, and onion, and stir-fry until tender-crisp.
5. Return the steak to the skillet.
6. Stir in soy sauce, oyster sauce, and the cornstarch mixture.
7. Cook for 2-3 minutes until the sauce has thickened.
8. Drizzle with sesame oil.
9. Serve immediately.

16. VEGETABLE STUFFED BELL PEPPERS

Ingredients:
- 4 bell peppers, tops cut off and seeds removed
- 1 cup cooked brown rice
- 1/2 cup black beans, rinsed and drained
- 1/2 cup corn kernels
- 1/2 cup diced tomatoes
- 1/4 cup diced onion
- 1 tbsp olive oil
- 1 tsp ground cumin
- 1 tsp chili powder
- Salt and pepper to taste

Instructions:
1. Preheat the oven to 375°F (190°C).
2. In a skillet, heat olive oil over medium heat.
3. Add onion and cook until softened.
4. Stir in rice, black beans, corn, tomatoes, cumin, chili powder, salt, and pepper.

5. Spoon the mixture into the bell pepper halves.
6. Place stuffed peppers in a baking dish and cover with foil.
7. Bake for 25-30 minutes, or until peppers are tender.
8. Serve warm.

17. HERB-CRUSTED PORK TENDERLOIN

Ingredients:
- 1 pork tenderloin (about 1 lb)
- 2 tbsp olive oil
- 1 tsp dried thyme
- 1 tsp dried rosemary
- 1 tsp garlic powder
- Salt and pepper to taste

Instructions:
1. Preheat the oven to 375°F (190°C).
2. In a small bowl, mix thyme, rosemary, garlic powder, salt, and pepper.
3. Rub the pork tenderloin with olive oil and coat with the herb mixture.
4. Place the tenderloin on a baking sheet.
5. Bake for 25-30 minutes, or until the internal temperature reaches 145°F (63°C).
6. Let the pork rest for 10 minutes before slicing.
7. Serve warm.

18. CHICKEN AND VEGETABLE CASSEROLE

Ingredients:
- 2 cups cooked, shredded chicken breast
- 1 cup broccoli florets
- 1 cup diced carrots
- 1/2 cup peas
- 1 cup low-sodium chicken broth
- 1/2 cup shredded cheddar cheese
- 1/2 cup whole wheat breadcrumbs

- 2 tbsp olive oil
- 1 tsp dried thyme
- Salt and pepper to taste

Instructions:
1. Preheat the oven to 375°F (190°C).
2. In a large bowl, combine chicken, broccoli, carrots, peas, chicken broth, thyme, salt, and pepper.
3. Transfer the mixture to a baking dish.
4. Top with shredded cheddar cheese and breadcrumbs.
5. Drizzle with olive oil.
6. Bake for 25-30 minutes, or until the top is golden brown and the vegetables are tender.
7. Serve warm.

19. GRILLED SALMON WITH AVOCADO SALSA

Ingredients:
- 2 salmon filets
- 1 tbsp olive oil
- 1 tsp ground cumin
- 1 tsp chili powder
- Salt and pepper to taste
- 1 avocado, diced
- 1/4 cup diced red onion
- 1/4 cup diced tomatoes
- 1 tbsp lime juice
- 1 tbsp chopped fresh cilantro

Instructions:
1. Preheat the grill to medium-high heat.
2. Rub salmon filets with olive oil, cumin, chili powder, salt, and pepper.
3. Grill the salmon for 4-5 minutes per side, or until cooked through.
4. In a small bowl, combine avocado, red onion, tomatoes, lime juice, and cilantro.

5. Serve the salmon topped with avocado salsa.

20. VEGETARIAN CHILI

Ingredients:
- 1 tbsp olive oil
- 1/2 cup diced onion
- 1/2 cup diced bell peppers
- 1/2 cup diced zucchini
- 1 cup diced tomatoes
- 1 cup black beans, rinsed and drained
- 1 cup kidney beans, rinsed and drained
- 2 cups vegetable broth
- 1 tbsp chili powder
- 1 tsp ground cumin
- 1 tsp smoked paprika
- Salt and pepper to taste

Instructions:
1. Heat olive oil in a large pot over medium heat.
2. Add onion and bell peppers, and sauté until softened.
3. Stir in zucchini, tomatoes, black beans, kidney beans, vegetable broth, chili powder, cumin, paprika, salt, and pepper.
4. Bring to a boil, then reduce heat and simmer for 25-30 minutes.
5. Serve hot.

6. Chapter 5: Snacks and Appetizers

1. HUMMUS AND VEGGIE PLATTER

Ingredients:
- 1 can chickpeas, drained and rinsed
- 2 tbsp tahini
- 2 tbsp lemon juice
- 2 cloves garlic, minced
- 1/4 cup olive oil
- 1/2 tsp cumin
- Salt to taste
- Assorted fresh vegetables (carrots, cucumbers, bell peppers, cherry tomatoes) for dipping

Instructions:
1. In a food processor, blend chickpeas, tahini, lemon juice, and garlic until smooth.
2. Slowly add olive oil while blending until desired consistency is reached.
3. Add cumin and salt to taste, blending well.
4. Serve with assorted fresh vegetables.

2. BAKED SWEET POTATO FRIES

Ingredients:
- 2 large sweet potatoes, peeled and cut into thin strips
- 2 tbsp olive oil
- 1 tsp paprika
- 1/2 tsp garlic powder
- Salt and pepper to taste

Instructions:
1. Preheat the oven to 425°F (220°C).

2. In a large bowl, toss sweet potato strips with olive oil, paprika, garlic powder, salt, and pepper.
3. Spread the sweet potato fries in a single layer on a baking sheet.
4. Bake for 20-25 minutes, turning halfway through, until crispy and golden.
5. Serve immediately.

3. CAPRESE SKEWERS

Ingredients:
- 1 pint cherry tomatoes
- 8 oz fresh mozzarella balls (bocconcini)
- Fresh basil leaves
- 2 tbsp balsamic glaze
- Wooden skewers

Instructions:
1. On each skewer, alternate cherry tomatoes, mozzarella balls, and basil leaves.
2. Arrange the skewers on a platter.
3. Drizzle with balsamic glaze before serving.

4. STUFFED MUSHROOMS

Ingredients:
- 1 lb button mushrooms, stems removed
- 1/2 cup whole wheat breadcrumbs
- 1/4 cup grated Parmesan cheese
- 2 cloves garlic, minced
- 2 tbsp fresh parsley, chopped
- 1/4 cup olive oil
- Salt and pepper to taste

Instructions:
1. Preheat the oven to 375°F (190°C).

2. In a bowl, combine breadcrumbs, Parmesan cheese, garlic, parsley, olive oil, salt, and pepper.
3. Fill each mushroom cap with the breadcrumb mixture.
4. Place stuffed mushrooms on a baking sheet.
5. Bake for 20 minutes, or until mushrooms are tender and tops are golden brown.
6. Serve warm.

5. GUACAMOLE

Ingredients:
- 3 ripe avocados
- 1 small onion, finely chopped
- 2 tomatoes, diced
- 1 jalapeño, seeded and minced
- 1/4 cup fresh cilantro, chopped
- 2 tbsp lime juice
- Salt to taste

Instructions:
1. In a bowl, mash the avocados until smooth.
2. Stir in onion, tomatoes, jalapeño, cilantro, lime juice, and salt.
3. Serve immediately with whole grain tortilla chips or fresh vegetables.

6. ROASTED CHICKPEAS

Ingredients:
- 1 can chickpeas, drained and rinscd
- 1 tbsp olive oil
- 1 tsp paprika
- 1/2 tsp garlic powder
- Salt and pepper to taste

Instructions:
1. Preheat the oven to 400°F (200°C).

2. In a bowl, toss chickpeas with olive oil, paprika, garlic powder, salt, and pepper.
3. Spread the chickpeas on a baking sheet in a single layer.
4. Roast for 25-30 minutes, stirring occasionally, until crispy.
5. Serve warm or at room temperature.

7. GREEK YOGURT AND CUCUMBER DIP

Ingredients:
- 1 cup Greek yogurt
- 1/2 cucumber, grated and drained
- 1 clove garlic, minced
- 1 tbsp fresh dill, chopped
- 1 tbsp lemon juice
- Salt and pepper to taste

Instructions:
1. In a bowl, combine Greek yogurt, grated cucumber, garlic, dill, lemon juice, salt, and pepper.
2. Mix well and refrigerate for at least 30 minutes before serving.
3. Serve with whole grain pita chips or fresh vegetables.

8. MINI QUICHE CUPS

Ingredients:
- 6 large eggs
- 1/4 cup milk
- 1/2 cup diced vegetables (spinach, bell peppers, mushrooms)
- 1/4 cup shredded cheese
- Salt and pepper to taste
- Non-stick cooking spray

Instructions:
1. Preheat the oven to 375°F (190°C).
2. In a mixing bowl, whisk together eggs, milk, salt, and pepper.

3. Stir in the diced vegetables and shredded cheese.
4. Spray a muffin tin with non-stick cooking spray.
5. Pour the egg mixture into the muffin cups, filling each about 3/4 full.
6. Bake for 20-25 minutes, or until the quiches are set and golden brown.
7. Let cool slightly before removing from the tin.
8. Serve warm or at room temperature.

9. DEVILED EGGS

Ingredients:
- 6 large eggs
- 3 tbsp Greek yogurt
- 1 tsp Dijon mustard
- 1 tsp apple cider vinegar
- Salt and pepper to taste
- Paprika for garnish

Instructions:
1. Place the eggs in a saucepan and cover with water. Bring to a boil over medium-high heat.
2. Once boiling, cover the saucepan, remove from heat, and let sit for 12 minutes.
3. Transfer the eggs to a bowl of ice water to cool.
4. Peel the eggs and cut them in half lengthwise.
5. Remove the yolks and place them in a bowl.
6. Mash the yolks with Greek yogurt, mustard, apple cider vinegar, salt, and pepper until smooth.
7. Spoon or pipe the yolk mixture back into the egg whites.
8. Sprinkle it with paprika before serving.

10. SPINACH AND FETA STUFFED MINI PEPPERS

Ingredients:
- 12 mini bell peppers, halved and seeded
- 1 cup fresh spinach, chopped

- 1/2 cup crumbled feta cheese
- 2 tbsp Greek yogurt
- 1 clove garlic, minced
- Salt and pepper to taste

Instructions:
1. Preheat the oven to 375°F (190°C).
2. In a bowl, combine spinach, feta cheese, Greek yogurt, garlic, salt, and pepper.
3. Fill each mini pepper half with the spinach and feta mixture.
4. Place stuffed peppers on a baking sheet.
5. Bake for 15-20 minutes, or until peppers are tender.
6. Serve warm.

11. CUCUMBER ROLLS WITH SMOKED SALMON

Ingredients:
- 1 large cucumber, thinly sliced lengthwise
- 4 oz smoked salmon, cut into strips
- 1/4 cup cream cheese
- 1 tbsp fresh dill, chopped
- 1 tbsp capers, rinsed and drained
- 1 tbsp lemon juice

Instructions:
1. In a bowl, combine cream cheese, dill, capers, and lemon juice.
2. Spread a thin layer of the cream cheese mixture on each cucumber slice.
3. Place a strip of smoked salmon at one end of each cucumber slice.
4. Roll up the cucumber slices and secure with toothpicks.
5. Serve immediately.

12. EDAMAME WITH SEA SALT

Ingredients:
- 2 cups edamame in pods

- 1 tbsp sea salt

Instructions:
1. Bring a pot of water to a boil.
2. Add the edamame pods and cook for 3-5 minutes until tender.
3. Drain and transfer to a bowl.
4. Sprinkle it with sea salt.
5. Serve warm.

13. TURKEY AND CHEESE PINWHEELS

Ingrcdicnts:
- 4 whole wheat tortillas
- 8 slices deli turkey
- 4 slices cheddar cheese
- 1/4 cup hummus
- Fresh spinach leaves

Instructions:
1. Spread hummus evenly over each tortilla.
2. Layer turkey slices, cheddar cheese, and spinach leaves on top.
3. Roll up the tortillas tightly.
4. Slice into 1-inch pinwheels.
5. Serve immediately or refrigerate until ready to serve.

14. BAKED ZUCCHINI CHIPS

Ingrcdicnts:
- 2 medium zucchinis, thinly sliced
- 1 tbsp olive oil
- 1/4 cup grated Parmesan cheese
- 1/2 tsp garlic powder
- Salt and pepper to taste

Instructions:

1. Preheat the oven to 425°F (220°C).
2. In a bowl, toss zucchini slices with olive oil, Parmesan cheese, garlic powder, salt, and pepper.
3. Arrange the zucchini slices in a single layer on a baking sheet.
4. Bake for 20-25 minutes, or until crispy and golden brown.
5. Serve immediately.

15. PEANUT BUTTER AND BANANA ROLL-UPS

Ingredients:
- 2 whole wheat tortillas
- 2 tbsp natural peanut butter
- 1 banana, sliced

Instructions:
1. Spread peanut butter evenly over each tortilla.
2. Arrange banana slices over the peanut butter.
3. Roll up the tortillas tightly.
4. Slice into 1-inch pieces.
5. Serve immediately or refrigerate until ready to serve.

16. PARMESAN KALE CHIPS

Ingredients:
- 1 bunch kale, stems removed and leaves torn into bite-sized pieces
- 1 tbsp olive oil
- 1/4 cup grated Parmesan cheese
- Salt and pepper to taste

Instructions:
1. Preheat the oven to 350°F (175°C).
2. In a bowl, toss kale leaves with olive oil, Parmesan cheese, salt, and pepper.
3. Spread the kale in a single layer on a baking sheet.

4. Bake for 10-15 minutes, or until crispy.

5. Serve immediately.

17. RICOTTA AND SPINACH STUFFED TOMATOES

Ingredients:
- 4 large tomatoes
- 1 cup ricotta cheese
- 1/2 cup fresh spinach, chopped
- 1 clove garlic, minced
- 1 tbsp fresh basil, chopped
- Salt and pepper to taste

Instructions:
1. Preheat the oven to 375°F (190°C).
2. Cut the tops off the tomatoes and scoop out the seeds and pulp.
3. In a bowl, combine ricotta cheese, spinach, garlic, basil, salt, and pepper.
4. Stuff the tomatoes with the ricotta mixture.
5. Place stuffed tomatoes on a baking sheet.
6. Bake for 20-25 minutes, or until tomatoes are tender.
7. Serve warm.

18. APPLE SLICES WITH ALMOND BUTTER

Ingredients:
- 2 apples, cored and sliced
- 1/4 cup almond butter

Instructions:
1. Arrange apple slices on a serving plate.
2. Serve with almond butter for dipping.

19. AVOCADO AND BLACK BEAN SALSA

Ingredients:
- 1 ripe avocado, diced
- 1 can black beans, drained and rinsed
- 1 small red onion, finely chopped
- 1 jalapeño, seeded and minced
- 1/4 cup fresh cilantro, chopped
- 2 tbsp lime juice
- Salt and pepper to taste

Instructions:
1. In a bowl, combine avocado, black beans, red onion, jalapeño, cilantro, lime juice, salt, and pepper.
2. Mix well and serve with whole grain tortilla chips or fresh vegetables.

20. ROASTED RED PEPPER HUMMUS

Ingredients:
- 1 can chickpeas, drained and rinsed
- 1 roasted red pepper, chopped
- 2 tbsp tahini
- 2 tbsp lemon juice
- 2 cloves garlic, minced
- 1/4 cup olive oil
- 1/2 tsp cumin
- Salt to taste

Instructions:
1. In a food processor, blend chickpeas, roasted red pepper, tahini, lemon juice, and garlic until smooth.
2. Slowly add olive oil while blending until desired consistency is reached.
3. Add cumin and salt to taste, blending well.
4. Serve with whole grain pita chips or fresh vegetables.

7. Chapter 6: Desserts

1. CHIA SEED PUDDING

Ingredients:
- 1/4 cup chia seeds
- 1 cup unsweetened almond milk
- 1 tbsp honey or maple syrup
- 1/2 tsp vanilla extract
- Fresh berries for topping

Instructions:
1. In a bowl, combine chia seeds, almond milk, honey or maple syrup, and vanilla extract.
2. Stir well and let sit for 5 minutes.
3. Stir again to prevent clumping.
4. Cover and refrigerate for at least 2 hours or overnight.
5. Top with fresh berries before serving.

2. BAKED APPLES

Ingredients:
- 4 large apples, cored
- 1/4 cup rolled oats
- 2 tbsp chopped nuts (walnuts or pecans)
- 2 tbsp raisins
- 1/2 tsp cinnamon
- 2 tbsp honey
- 1/4 cup water

Instructions:
1. Preheat the oven to 350°F (175°C).
2. In a bowl, combine oats, nuts, raisins, cinnamon, and honey.
3. Stuff the mixture into the cored apples.

4. Place the apples in a baking dish and add water to the dish.
5. Bake for 30-40 minutes, or until the apples are tender.
6. Serve warm.

3. YOGURT PARFAIT

Ingredients:
- 2 cups Greek yogurt
- 1 cup granola
- 1 cup mixed berries (strawberries, blueberries, raspberries)
- 2 tbsp honey

Instructions:
1. In serving glasses, layer Greek yogurt, granola, and mixed berries.
2. Drizzle with honey.
3. Repeat layers and serve immediately.

4. BANANA ICE CREAM

Ingredients:
- 3 ripe bananas, sliced and frozen
- 1 tsp vanilla extract
- Optional toppings: chopped nuts, dark chocolate shavings, fresh berries

Instructions:
1. In a food processor, blend frozen banana slices until smooth and creamy.
2. Add vanilla extract and blend until combined.
3. Serve immediately with optional toppings.

5. PEAR CRISP

Ingredients:
- 4 ripe pears, peeled and sliced
- 1/2 cup rolled oats
- 1/4 cup almond flour

- 1/4 cup chopped nuts (walnuts or pecans)
- 1/4 cup honey
- 1 tsp cinnamon
- 2 tbsp coconut oil, melted

Instructions:
1. Preheat the oven to 350°F (175°C).
2. Place pear slices in a baking dish.
3. In a bowl, combine oats, almond flour, nuts, honey, cinnamon, and melted coconut oil.
4. Sprinkle the oat mixture over the pears.
5. Bake for 25-30 minutes, or until the top is golden brown and the pears are tender.
6. Serve warm.

6. CHOCOLATE AVOCADO MOUSSE

Ingredients:
- 2 ripe avocados
- 1/4 cup cocoa powder
- 1/4 cup honey or maple syrup
- 1/2 tsp vanilla extract
- Pinch of salt

Instructions:
1. In a food processor, blend avocados until smooth.
2. Add cocoa powder, honey or maple syrup, vanilla extract, and salt.
3. Blend until well combined and smooth.
4. Serve immediately or chill before serving.

7. OATMEAL COOKIES

Ingredients:
- 1 cup rolled oats
- 1/2 cup almond flour

- 1/4 cup honey
- 1/4 cup coconut oil, melted
- 1/2 tsp cinnamon
- 1/4 cup raisins
- 1/4 cup chopped nuts (walnuts or pecans)

Instructions:
1. Preheat the oven to 350°F (175°C).
2. In a bowl, combine oats, almond flour, honey, coconut oil, cinnamon, raisins, and nuts.
3. Drop spoonfuls of dough onto a baking sheet lined with parchment paper.
4. Flatten slightly with the back of a spoon.
5. Bake for 10-12 minutes, or until golden brown.
6. Cool on a wire rack before serving.

8. MANGO SORBET

Ingredients:
- 2 ripe mangoes, peeled and chopped
- 1/4 cup water
- 2 tbsp honey or maple syrup
- 1 tbsp lime juice

Instructions:
1. In a blender, puree mangoes, water, honey or maple syrup, and lime juice until smooth.
2. Pour the mixture into a shallow dish and freeze for at least 2 hours.
3. Scrape with a fork to create a slushy texture before serving.

9. RICOTTA AND BERRY DESSERT

Ingredients:
- 1 cup ricotta cheese
- 1 tbsp honey

- 1/2 tsp vanilla extract
- 1 cup mixed berries (strawberries, blueberries, raspberries)

Instructions:
1. In a bowl, combine ricotta cheese, honey, and vanilla extract.
2. Spoon the ricotta mixture into serving dishes.
3. Top with mixed berries.
4. Serve immediately.

10. COCONUT MACAROONS

Ingredients:
- 2 cups shredded unsweetened coconut
- 1/2 cup almond flour
- 1/4 cup honey
- 1/4 cup coconut oil, melted
- 1/2 tsp vanilla extract
- Pinch of salt

Instructions:
1. Preheat the oven to 325°F (165°C).
2. In a bowl, combine shredded coconut, almond flour, honey, melted coconut oil, vanilla extract, and salt.
3. Drop spoonfuls of the mixture onto a baking sheet lined with parchment paper.
4. Bake for 15-20 minutes, or until golden brown.
5. Cool on a wire rack before serving.

11. PEACH AND BLUEBERRY COBBLER

Ingredients:
- 4 ripe peaches, peeled and sliced
- 1 cup blueberries
- 1/4 cup honey
- 1 cup almond flour

- 1/2 cup rolled oats
- 1/4 cup coconut oil, melted
- 1 tsp cinnamon

Instructions:
1. Preheat the oven to 350°F (175°C).
2. In a baking dish, combine peaches, blueberries, and honey.
3. In a bowl, combine almond flour, rolled oats, coconut oil, and cinnamon.
4. Sprinkle the oat mixture over the fruit.
5. Bake for 25-30 minutes, or until the top is golden brown and the fruit is bubbly.
6. Serve warm.

12. STRAWBERRY BANANA SMOOTHIE

Ingredients:
- 1 cup strawberries, hulled and sliced
- 1 ripe banana
- 1 cup unsweetened almond milk
- 1 tbsp honey or maple syrup
- 1/2 tsp vanilla extract

Instructions:
1. In a blender, combine strawberries, banana, almond milk, honey or maple syrup, and vanilla extract.
2. Blend until smooth.
3. Serve immediately.

13. APPLE CINNAMON ENERGY BALLS

Ingredients:
- 1 cup rolled oats
- 1/2 cup almond butter
- 1/4 cup honey
- 1/2 cup dried apples, chopped

- 1 tsp cinnamon

Instructions:
1. In a bowl, combine rolled oats, almond butter, honey, dried apples, and cinnamon.
2. Mix well until combined.
3. Roll into bite-sized balls.
4. Refrigerate for at least 30 minutes before serving.

14. BAKED PEACHES WITH HONEY AND ALMONDS

Ingredients:
- 4 ripe peaches, halved and pitted
- 2 tbsp honey
- 1/4 cup sliced almonds
- 1/2 tsp cinnamon

Instructions:
1. Preheat the oven to 350°F (175°C).
2. Place peach halves in a baking dish.
3. Drizzle with honey and sprinkle with sliced almonds and cinnamon.
4. Bake for 20-25 minutes, or until peaches are tender.
5. Serve warm.

15. PINEAPPLE COCONUT BARS

Ingredients:
- 1 1/2 cups almond flour
- 1/4 cup coconut oil, melted
- 1/4 cup honey
- 1/2 cup crushed pineapple, drained
- 1/4 cup shredded unsweetened coconut

Instructions:
1. Preheat the oven to 350°F (175°C).

2. In a bowl, combine almond flour, melted coconut oil, and honey.

3. Press the mixture into a baking dish to form a crust.

4. Spread crushed pineapple over the crust and sprinkle with shredded coconut.

5. Bake for 20-25 minutes, or until the edges are golden brown.

6. Cool completely before cutting into bars.

16. AVOCADO LIME CHEESECAKE

Ingredients:
- 2 ripe avocados
- 1/4 cup lime juice
- 1/4 cup honey
- 1 cup Greek yogurt
- 1 tsp vanilla extract
- 1 pre-made graham cracker crust

Instructions:

1. In a blender, combine avocados, lime juice, honey, Greek yogurt, and vanilla extract.

2. Blend until smooth and creamy.

33. Pour the avocado mixture into the pre-made graham cracker crust.

4. Smooth the top with a spatula.

5. Refrigerate for at least 2 hours before serving.

6. Garnish with lime zest if desired.

17. BERRY COMPOTE WITH GREEK YOGURT

Ingredients:
- 1 cup mixed berries (strawberries, blueberries, raspberries)
- 2 tbsp honey
- 1/4 cup water
- 2 cups Greek yogurt

Instructions:
1. In a saucepan, combine mixed berries, honey, and water.
2. Bring to a simmer over medium heat and cook for 5-7 minutes, or until the berries are soft and the sauce has thickened.
3. Let the berry compote cool slightly.
4. Spoon Greek yogurt into serving bowls and top with the berry compote.
5. Serve immediately.

18. CINNAMON BAKED PEARS

Ingredients:
- 4 ripe pears, halved and cored
- 2 tbsp honey
- 1/2 tsp cinnamon
- 1/4 cup chopped walnuts

Instructions:
1. Preheat the oven to 350°F (175°C).
2. Place pear halves in a baking dish.
3. Drizzle with honey and sprinkle with cinnamon and chopped walnuts.
4. Bake for 20-25 minutes, or until the pears are tender.
5. Serve warm.

19. COCONUT MILK RICE PUDDING

Ingredients:
- 1 cup cooked brown rice
- 1 cup coconut milk
- 1/4 cup honey or maple syrup
- 1/2 tsp vanilla extract
- 1/4 cup shredded unsweetened coconut
- 1/4 tsp cinnamon

Instructions:
1. In a saucepan, combine cooked brown rice, coconut milk, honey or maple syrup, and vanilla extract.
2. Cook over medium heat, stirring frequently, until the mixture thickens, about 10 minutes.
3. Stir in shredded coconut and cinnamon.
4. Serve warm or chilled.

20. LEMON POPPY SEED MUFFINS

Ingredients:
- 1 1/2 cups almond flour
- 1/4 cup coconut flour
- 1/4 cup honey
- 1/4 cup coconut oil, melted
- 3 eggs
- 1/4 cup lemon juice
- 1 tbsp lemon zest
- 1 tbsp poppy seeds
- 1/2 tsp baking soda
- 1/4 tsp salt

Instructions:
1. Preheat the oven to 350°F (175°C).
2. In a bowl, combine almond flour, coconut flour, honey, melted coconut oil, eggs, lemon juice, lemon zest, poppy seeds, baking soda, and salt.
3. Mix until well combined.
4. Divide the batter evenly among a greased muffin tin.
5. Bake for 18-20 minutes, or until a toothpick inserted into the center comes out clean.
6. Cool on a wire rack before serving.

8. Chapter 7: Beverages

1. CUCUMBER MINT WATER

Ingredients:
- 1 cucumber, thinly sliced
- 10 fresh mint leaves
- 8 cups water
- Ice cubes

Instructions:
1. In a large pitcher, combine cucumber slices, mint leaves, and water.
2. Stir well and refrigerate for at least 2 hours to let the flavors infuse.
3. Serve over ice.

2. GINGER LEMON TEA

Ingredients:
- 1-inch piece fresh ginger, peeled and sliced
- 1 lemon, sliced
- 4 cups water
- Honey to taste

Instructions:
1. In a saucepan, bring water to a boil.
2. Add ginger and lemon slices.
3. Reduce heat and simmer for 10 minutes.
4. Strain the tea into mugs and sweeten with honey to taste.
5. Serve warm.

3. BLUEBERRY SMOOTHIE

Ingredients:
- 1 cup fresh or frozen blueberries

- 1 banana
- 1 cup unsweetened almond milk
- 1 tbsp honey or maple syrup
- 1/2 tsp vanilla extract

Instructions:
1. In a blender, combine blueberries, banana, almond milk, honey or maple syrup, and vanilla extract.
2. Blend until smooth.
3. Serve immediately.

4. TURMERIC LATTE

Ingredients:
- 1 cup unsweetened almond milk
- 1/2 tsp ground turmeric
- 1/4 tsp ground cinnamon
- 1/4 tsp ground ginger
- 1 tbsp honey or maple syrup
- Pinch of black pepper

Instructions:
1. In a small saucepan, heat almond milk over medium heat until warm.
2. Whisk in turmeric, cinnamon, ginger, honey or maple syrup, and black pepper.
3. Continue to whisk until well combined and frothy.
4. Serve warm.

5. SPINACH AND APPLE SMOOTHIE

Ingredients:
- 1 cup fresh spinach
- 1 apple, cored and chopped
- 1 banana
- 1 cup unsweetened almond milk

- 1 tbsp honey or maple syrup

Instructions:
1. In a blender, combine spinach, apple, banana, almond milk, and honey or
maple syrup.
2. Blend until smooth.
3. Serve immediately.

6. CINNAMON APPLE CIDER

Ingredients:
- 4 cups apple cider
- 2 cinnamon sticks
- 1/2 tsp ground cloves
- 1/4 tsp ground nutmeg

Instructions:
1. In a saucepan, combine apple cider, cinnamon sticks, ground cloves, and
ground nutmeg.
2. Bring to a simmer over medium heat.
3. Reduce heat and simmer for 10 minutes.
4. Serve warm.

7. WATERMELON COOLER

Ingredients:
- 4 cups cubed watermelon
- 1 cup water
- Juice of 1 lime
- Fresh mint leaves for garnish

Instructions:
1. In a blender, combine watermelon, water, and lime juice.
2. Blend until smooth.
3. Serve over ice and garnish with fresh mint leaves.

8. CARROT ORANGE JUICE

Ingredients:
- 4 large carrots, peeled and chopped
- 2 oranges, peeled and segmented
- 1-inch piece fresh ginger, peeled and sliced

Instructions:
1. In a juicer, process carrots, oranges, and ginger.
2. Stir well and serve immediately.

9. STRAWBERRY BASIL LEMONADE

Ingredients:
- 1 cup fresh strawberries, hulled and sliced
- 1/4 cup fresh basil leaves
- 1/2 cup lemon juice
- 4 cups water
- 1/4 cup honey

Instructions:
1. In a blender, combine strawberries, basil leaves, lemon juice, and honey.
2. Blend until smooth.
3. Strain the mixture through a fine mesh sieve into a pitcher.
4. Add water and stir well.
5. Serve over ice.

10. PEAR AND SPINACH SMOOTHIE

Ingredients:
- 1 ripe pear, cored and chopped
- 1 cup fresh spinach
- 1 banana
- 1 cup unsweetened almond milk
- 1 tbsp honey or maple syrup

Instructions:
1. In a blender, combine pear, spinach, banana, almond milk, and honey or maple syrup.
2. Blend until smooth.
3. Serve immediately.

11. POMEGRANATE GREEN TEA

Ingredients:
- 2 cups water
- 2 green tea bags
- 1/2 cup pomegranate juice
- 1 tbsp honey

Instructions:
1. In a saucepan, bring water to a boil.
2. Remove from heat and steep green tea bags for 3-5 minutes.
3. Remove tea bags and stir in pomegranate juice and honey.
4. Serve warm or over ice.

12. MANGO LASSI

Ingredients:
- 1 cup fresh or frozen mango chunks
- 1 cup Greek yogurt
- 1/2 cup water
- 1 tbsp honey or maple syrup
- 1/4 tsp ground cardamom

Instructions:
1. In a blender, combine mango, Greek yogurt, water, honey or maple syrup, and ground cardamom.
2. Blend until smooth.
3. Serve immediately.

13. PEACH GINGER ICED TEA

Ingredients:
- 4 cups water
- 2 black tea bags
- 1 ripe peach, sliced
- 1-inch piece fresh ginger, peeled and sliced
- 1/4 cup honey

Instructions:
1. In a saucepan, bring water to a boil.
2. Remove from heat and steep black tea bags for 3-5 minutes.
3. Remove tea bags and add peach slices, ginger, and honey.
4. Let the mixture cool to room temperature.
5. Strain and serve over ice.

14. CUCUMBER LEMON DETOX WATER

Ingredients:
- 1 cucumber, thinly sliced
- 1 lemon, thinly sliced
- 8 cups water
- Ice cubes

Instructions:
1. In a large pitcher, combine cucumber slices, lemon slices, and water.
2. Stir well and refrigerate for at least 2 hours to let the flavors infuse.
3. Serve over ice.

15. PINEAPPLE COCONUT SMOOTHIE

Ingredients:
- 1 cup fresh or frozen pineapple chunks
- 1/2 cup coconut milk
- 1/2 cup unsweetened almond milk

- 1 tbsp honey or maple syrup

Instructions:
1. In a blender, combine pineapple, coconut milk, almond milk, and honey or maple syrup.
2. Blend until smooth.
3. Serve immediately.

16. BEETROOT APPLE JUICE

Ingredients:
- 2 medium beetroots, peeled and chopped
- 2 apples, cored and chopped
- 1-inch piece fresh ginger, peeled and sliced

Instructions:
1. In a juicer, process beetroots, apples, and ginger.
2. Stir well and serve immediately.

17. ORANGE CREAMSICLE SMOOTHIE

Ingredients:
- 2 oranges, peeled and segmented
- 1/2 cup Greek yogurt
- 1/2 cup unsweetened almond milk
- 1 tbsp honey or maple syrup
- 1/2 tsp vanilla extract

Instructions:
1. In a blender, combine oranges, Greek yogurt, almond milk, honey or maple syrup, and vanilla extract.
2. Blend until smooth.
3. Serve immediately.

18. MINTY GREEN JUICE

Ingredients:
- 1 cucumber, peeled and chopped
- 1 green apple, cored and chopped
- 1 cup fresh spinach
- 1/2 cup fresh mint leaves
- 1/2 lemon, juiced

Instructions:
1. In a juicer, process cucumber, green apple, spinach, and mint leaves.
2. Stir in lemon juice.
3. Serve immediately.

19. SPICED APPLE CIDER

Ingredients:
- 4 cups apple cider
- 2 cinnamon sticks
- 1/2 tsp ground allspice
- 1/4 tsp ground cloves

Instructions:
1. In a saucepan, combine apple cider, cinnamon sticks, ground allspice, and ground cloves.
2. Bring to a simmer over medium heat.
3. Reduce heat and simmer for 10 minutes.
4. Serve warm.

20. BERRY DETOX SMOOTHIE

Ingredients:
- 1 cup mixed berries (strawberries, blueberries, raspberries)
- 1 cup unsweetened almond milk
- 1 tbsp honey or maple syrup

- 1 tbsp chia seeds

Instructions:
1. In a blender, combine mixed berries, almond milk, honey or maple syrup, and chia seeds.
2. Blend until smooth.
3. Serve immediately.

9. Chapter 8: 7-Day Meal Plan

Day 1
Breakfast:
- Oatmeal with Fresh Berries
- Herbal Tea

Lunch:
- Grilled Chicken Salad with Spinach and Strawberries
- Cucumber Mint Water

Dinner:
- Baked Salmon with Steamed Asparagus and Quinoa
- Lemon Ginger Tea

Snack:
- Apple Slices with Almond Butter

Dessert:
- Coconut Milk Rice Pudding

Day 2
Breakfast:
- Greek Yogurt with Honey and Walnuts
- Blueberry Smoothie

Lunch:
- Turkey and Avocado Wrap with Mixed Greens
- Watermelon Cooler

Dinner:
- Stuffed Bell Peppers with Ground Turkey and Brown Rice
- Cinnamon Apple Cider

Snack:
- Carrot Sticks with Hummus

Dessert:
- Lemon Poppy Seed Muffins

 Day 3
Breakfast:
- Spinach and Feta Omelette
- Ginger Lemon Tea

Lunch:
- Lentil and Vegetable Soup
- Cucumber Lemon Detox Water

Dinner:
- Herb-Roasted Chicken with Steamed Broccoli and Sweet Potato
- Pomegranate Green Tea

Snack:
- Celery Sticks with Low-Sodium Cottage Cheese

Dessert:
- Avocado Lime Pie

 Day 4
Breakfast:
- Chia Seed Pudding with Fresh Mango
- Minty Green Juice

Lunch:
- Quinoa Salad with Roasted Vegetables
- Peach Ginger Iced Tea

Dinner:
- Baked Cod with Tomato Basil Sauce and Green Beans
- Spiced Apple Cider

Snack:
- Pear and Spinach Smoothie

Dessert:
- Baked Apples with Cinnamon and Walnuts

Day 5
Breakfast:
- Whole Wheat Toast with Mashed Avocado and Tomato Slices
- Orange Creamsicle Smoothie

Lunch:
- Chicken and Vegetable Stir-Fry
- Berry Detox Smoothie

Dinner:
- Grilled Shrimp with Zucchini Noodles
- Turmeric Latte

Snack:
- Mixed Nuts and Dried Fruit

Dessert:
- Strawberry Basil Lemonade Sorbet

Day 6
Breakfast:
- Smoothie Bowl with Bananas, Berries, and Chia Seeds
- Pineapple Coconut Smoothie

Lunch:
- Black Bean and Corn Salad with Lime Dressing
- Beetroot Apple Juice

Dinner:
- Turkey Meatballs with Spaghetti Squash
- Lemon Water

Snack:
- Sliced Bell Peppers with Guacamole

Dessert:
- Berry Compote with Greek Yogurt

 Day 7
Breakfast:
- Whole Grain Pancakes with Fresh Berries
- Spinach and Apple Smoothie

Lunch:
- Salmon and Avocado Salad with Lemon Dressing
- Watermelon Cooler

Dinner:
- Vegetable Stir-Fry with Tofu
- Cucumber Mint Water

Snack:
- Rice Cakes with Almond Butter

Dessert:
- Cinnamon Baked Pears

- **Grocery Shopping List for 7-Day Meal Plan**

Produce
- Apples (6)
- Asparagus (1 bunch)
- Avocados (5)
- Bananas (3)
- Bell Peppers (4)
- Blueberries (1 pint)
- Broccoli (1 head)
- Carrots (1 bunch)
- Celery (1 bunch)
- Chia Seeds (1 small bag)
- Cucumber (3)
- Fresh Basil (1 small bunch)
- Fresh Ginger (1 piece)
- Fresh Mint (1 small bunch)
- Fresh Spinach (2 bags)
- Garlic (1 head)
- Green Beans (1 pound)
- Green Apple (1)
- Lemon (6)
- Mixed Berries (1 bag frozen or fresh)
- Mixed Nuts and Dried Fruit (1 small bag)
- Oranges (6)
- Pears (5)
- Pineapple (1)
- Quinoa (1 small bag)
- Raspberries (1 pint)
- Strawberries (2 pints)
- Sweet Potatoes (2)
- Tomatoes (4)
- Zucchini (3)
- Strawberries (1 pint)

Dairy/Alternatives
- Almond Milk (1 carton)
- Coconut Milk (1 can)
- Greek Yogurt (1 large container)
- Low-Sodium Cottage Cheese (1 container)
- Unsweetened Almond Milk (1 carton)

Meat/Protein
- Baked Cod (1 filet)
- Baked Salmon (1 filet)
- Chicken Breasts (4)
- Chicken Thighs (2)
- Eggs (1 dozen)
- Ground Turkey (1 pound)
- Shrimp (1 pound)
- Turkey Meatballs (1 bag frozen or fresh)
- Tofu (1 package)
- Grilled Chicken (1 breast)
- Herb-Roasted Chicken (1 whole or parts)
- Grilled Shrimp (1 pound)

Grains
- Brown Rice (1 bag)
- Oatmeal (1 container)
- Whole Grain Pancake Mix (1 box)
- Whole Wheat Toast (1 loaf)
- Whole Wheat Wraps (1 package)

Spices and Condiments
- Black Pepper
- Cinnamon
- Ground Cardamom
- Ground Cloves
- Ground Ginger
- Ground Nutmeg

- Ground Turmeric
- Honey
- Lemon Zest (from lemons)
- Maple Syrup
- Olive Oil
- Poppy Seeds
- Salt
- Tomato Basil Sauce (1 jar)

 Beverages
- Apple Cider (1 carton)
- Green Tea Bags (1 box)
- Herbal Tea (1 box)
- Pomegranate Juice (1 bottle)

 Snacks and Desserts
- Almond Butter (1 jar)
- Graham Cracker Crust (1 pre-made)
- Hummus (1 container)
- Mixed Nuts and Dried Fruit (1 small bag)
- Rice Cakes (1 package)
- Sorbet (1 container)

This list covers all the ingredients needed for the 7-day meal plan, ensuring a variety of healthy and kidney-friendly meals.

- **Meal Prep Tips**

1. Consult with a Healthcare Professional
   - Always consult with your doctor or a registered dietitian before starting any new diet plan. They can provide personalized recommendations based on your specific health needs.

2. Focus on Fresh Produce
   - Incorporate plenty of fresh fruits and vegetables into your meals. These are generally low in sodium and high in essential nutrients. However, be mindful of potassium and phosphorus content, as certain fruits and vegetables can be high in these minerals.

3. Limit Sodium Intake
   - Choose fresh foods over processed ones, as processed foods often contain high levels of sodium. Season your food with herbs and spices instead of salt to add flavor without increasing sodium intake.

4. Control Protein Portions
   - While protein is essential, too much can put a strain on your kidneys. Focus on lean protein sources like chicken, turkey, fish, and plant-based proteins, and monitor portion sizes.

5. Monitor Potassium and Phosphorus
   - Some people with kidney disease need to limit foods high in potassium and phosphorus. Examples include bananas, oranges, potatoes, and dairy products. Work with your dietitian to identify the right balance for you.

6. Stay Hydrated
   - Proper hydration is crucial, but fluid intake may need to be controlled depending on your specific condition. Follow your healthcare provider's guidelines on how much fluid you should consume daily.

7. Plan and Prepare Meals Ahead
   - Planning and preparing meals in advance can help you stick to your diet and avoid unhealthy food choices. Consider preparing large batches and freezing portions for convenience.

8. Read Food Labels
   - Get into the habit of reading food labels to check for sodium, potassium, and phosphorus content. This is especially important for packaged and processed foods.

9. Balance Your Meals
   - Ensure each meal includes a variety of food groups: lean proteins, whole grains, fruits, and vegetables. This balance helps provide essential nutrients while managing kidney health.

10. Limit Phosphorus Additives
   - Phosphorus additives are often found in processed foods and beverages. These additives are easily absorbed by the body and can be harmful to people with kidney disease. Look for ingredient lists that mention "phos-" to identify these additives.

11. Use Healthy Cooking Methods
   - Opt for baking, grilling, steaming, and sautéing instead of frying. These methods help retain nutrients and reduce unhealthy fats in your meals.

12. Incorporate Healthy Fats
   - Include sources of healthy fats in your diet, such as olive oil, avocados, nuts, and seeds. These can help improve heart health, which is important for kidney disease patients.

13. Watch Out for Hidden Sodium
   - Be aware of hidden sodium in foods like canned vegetables, soups, and condiments. Choose low-sodium or no-salt-added versions when possible.

14. Maintain a Food Journal

   - Keeping a food journal can help you track what you eat and ensure you're following your meal plan. It can also help identify any foods that may cause issues.

15. Stay Active

  - Combine your healthy eating plan with regular physical activity. Exercise can help improve overall health and well-being.

By following these tips, you can better manage stage 3 kidney disease through a balanced and thoughtful diet, promoting overall health and well-being.

10. **Chapter 9: Tips for Dining Out**

Dining out can be a pleasurable experience, but for those managing Stage 3 kidney disease, it can also present some challenges. With careful planning and informed choices, you can enjoy meals at restaurants while adhering to your dietary needs. Here are some practical tips to help you dine out safely and enjoyably.

1. Research the Menu in Advance
   - Plan Ahead: Look up the restaurant's menu online before you go. This allows you to identify kidney-friendly options and avoid last-minute, potentially unhealthy choices.
   - Call Ahead: If the menu isn't detailed online, don't hesitate to call the restaurant and ask about their dishes. Inquire about ingredients and how dishes are prepared.

2. Communicate Your Dietary Needs
   - Inform the Staff: When you arrive, inform your server about your dietary restrictions due to kidney disease. Most restaurants are willing to accommodate special requests.
   - Ask Questions: Don't be shy about asking how dishes are prepared and if they can be modified to meet your needs, such as reducing salt or using fresh ingredients.

3. Choose Kidney-Friendly Dishes
   - Opt for Fresh Ingredients: Select dishes that emphasize fresh vegetables, lean proteins, and whole grains. Avoid dishes with heavy sauces, cheeses, and high-sodium ingredients.
   - Grilled, Baked, or Steamed: Choose cooking methods like grilling, baking, or steaming over frying to reduce unhealthy fats and sodium.

4. Control Portions
   - Share Dishes: Restaurant portions are often large. Consider sharing an entrée with a dining companion or ask for a half-portion if available.

- Take Leftovers Home: If the portion is too large, eat a reasonable amount and take the rest home for another meal. This can help you avoid overeating.

5. Limit High-Sodium Foods
   - Avoid Processed Foods: Steer clear of processed meats, salty appetizers, and canned soups, which are typically high in sodium.
   - Request No Added Salt: Ask the kitchen to prepare your food without added salt. Use herbs, lemon, or pepper to enhance the flavor instead.

6. Be Cautious with Sauces and Dressings
   - On the Side: Request sauces, dressings, and gravies on the side so you can control the amount you use.
   - Opt for Oil and Vinegar: Choose oil and vinegar for salads instead of creamy or commercial dressings, which can be high in sodium and phosphates.

7. Mind Your Beverages
   - Avoid High-Sodium Beverages: Stay away from tomato juice, certain sports drinks, and other high-sodium beverages.
   - Hydrate Wisely: Stick to water, herbal teas, or other low-sodium beverages. Avoid excessive alcohol, as it can affect your kidneys and overall health.

8. Choose Wisely with Sides
   - Healthy Sides: Opt for sides like steamed vegetables, salads, or baked potatoes without butter and sour cream. Avoid fries, mashed potatoes with gravy, and other high-sodium sides.
   - Custom Sides: If possible, request plain rice, quinoa, or another whole grain as a side dish.

9. Special Dietary Menus

- Seek Special Menus: Some restaurants offer menus specifically for people with dietary restrictions. Ask if they have a low-sodium or heart-healthy menu.

   - Chain Restaurants: Many chain restaurants have nutrition information available, making it easier to choose kidney-friendly options.

10. Desserts in Moderation

   - Fruit-Based Desserts: Opt for fresh fruit, fruit sorbet, or other light desserts instead of heavy, rich options like cake or pie.

   - Skip the Extras: Avoid toppings like whipped cream, caramel, and chocolate sauce, which can add unnecessary sugar and sodium.

11. Plan Your Day

   - Balance Your Meals: If you know you'll be dining out for dinner, plan lighter, kidney-friendly meals for breakfast and lunch. This helps balance your overall intake for the day.

   - Adjust Fluid Intake: Monitor your fluid intake throughout the day to account for beverages you might consume while dining out.

Dining out with Stage 3 kidney disease requires a bit of extra planning and communication, but with these tips, you can enjoy a meal at a restaurant without compromising your dietary needs. Remember to stay informed, ask questions, and make choices that align with your health goals.

11. Chapter 10: Managing Special Occasions

Special occasions such as holidays, family gatherings, and celebrations often revolve around food and can pose challenges for those managing Stage 3 kidney disease. However, with thoughtful planning and a few strategies, you can enjoy these events while keeping your health in check. Here's how to navigate special occasions without compromising your dietary needs.

1. Plan Ahead
   - Know the Menu: If possible, find out what will be served in advance. This allows you to plan your meals for the day and ensure you have suitable options available.
   - Bring a Dish: Offer to bring a kidney-friendly dish to share. This guarantees there will be something you can eat and introduces others to healthy eating options.

2. Portion Control
   - Small Servings: Opt for small servings of different foods to enjoy a variety without overeating. This is especially useful when faced with a buffet or multiple-course meal.
   - Mindful Eating: Eat slowly and savor each bite. This can help you feel fuller and more satisfied, making it easier to control portions.

3. Healthy Choices
   - Focus on Vegetables: Fill most of your plate with vegetables, but be mindful of those high in potassium and phosphorus. Opt for lower-potassium options like green beans, carrots, and cauliflower.
   - Lean Proteins: Choose lean protein sources such as turkey, chicken, or fish. Avoid high-sodium meats like ham or processed sausages.

4. Limit Sodium and Potassium

- Season Wisely: Avoid dishes with high sodium content, such as those with soy sauce, canned soups, or processed meats. Instead, opt for foods seasoned with herbs and spices.

- Watch High-Potassium Foods: Be cautious with high-potassium foods like potatoes, tomatoes, and certain fruits. If these are staples at the event, consume them in moderation.

5. Stay Hydrated

- Drink Water: Keep a water bottle with you and sip throughout the event. Staying hydrated can help manage your overall fluid balance.

- Avoid Sugary Drinks: Limit sugary beverages and alcohol, as they can add unnecessary calories and affect your hydration.

6. Communicate Your Needs

- Talk to the Host: Let the host know about your dietary restrictions in advance. Most hosts will appreciate your openness and be willing to accommodate your needs.

- Ask Questions: Don't hesitate to ask about ingredients and preparation methods of the dishes served. This helps you make informed choices.

7. Moderate Indulgence

- Treat Yourself Carefully: It's okay to indulge a little, but do so mindfully. Opt for smaller portions of your favorite treats and balance them with healthier options.

- Skip the Extras: Avoid extra toppings like gravy, butter, or heavy sauces that can add sodium and fats.

8. Stay Active

- Move Around: Engage in light physical activities before and after meals to help with digestion and maintain overall well-being.

- Socialize: Focus on the social aspects of the event rather than just the food. Enjoy conversations, games, and activities with friends and family.

9. Manage Stress

- Relax: Special occasions can be stressful. Practice deep breathing, meditation, or other relaxation techniques to keep stress levels down, which can benefit your overall health.

   - Enjoy the Moment: Focus on the joy of the occasion and the company of loved ones rather than worrying too much about dietary restrictions.

10. Post-Event Recovery
   - Hydrate Well: After the event, ensure you drink plenty of water to help flush out any excess sodium.

   - Healthy Meals: Return to your regular, kidney-friendly diet as soon as possible. Incorporate lots of fresh vegetables, lean proteins, and whole grains to balance out any indulgences.

   - Monitor Your Health: Keep an eye on how your body responds after special occasions. If you notice any adverse effects, consult your healthcare provider.

Sample Kidney-Friendly Dishes for Special Occasions

Here are some kidney-friendly dishes you can prepare and bring to special occasions:

Appetizer:
- Fresh Veggie Platter with Hummus
   - A colorful assortment of bell peppers, cucumbers, carrots, and celery served with a low-sodium hummus.

Main Dish:
- Herb-Roasted Chicken
   - Chicken breast seasoned with rosemary, thyme, and lemon, roasted to perfection.

Side Dish:
- Quinoa Salad with Vegetables
   - Quinoa mixed with diced cucumbers, bell peppers, and fresh herbs, dressed with a light lemon vinaigrette.

Dessert:
- Baked Apples with Cinnamon
  - Apples baked with a sprinkle of cinnamon and a touch of honey, served warm.

Special occasions are meant to be enjoyed. With these tips and a bit of preparation, you can partake in the celebrations while maintaining your kidney health. Remember, the goal is to enjoy the moment and make memories with your loved ones while staying mindful of your dietary needs.

13. Conclusion

In conclusion, managing Stage 3 kidney disease doesn't mean you have to miss out on special occasions or dining out. With careful planning, smart choices, and open communication, you can enjoy these events while keeping your health in check.

Remember to focus on fresh, whole foods, control portions, and limit sodium and potassium intake. Stay hydrated, stay active, and be mindful of your stress levels. Most importantly, don't be afraid to advocate for your dietary needs and ask questions when dining out or attending special occasions.

By following these tips and staying proactive about your health, you can continue to enjoy life's celebrations while managing your kidney health effectively. Here's to your health and happiness!